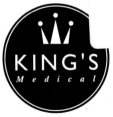

KING'S
Medical

KING'S

GUIDE to TENS

A User's Guide to

Transcutaneous Electrical

Nerve Stimulation

Alan King

Grad. Dip. Phys. MCSP SRP

Design and illustrations by
David J. Elliott

ISBN 0-9535623-0-1
Published by Kings Medical
Revised Edition .

c o n t e n t s

Introduction

THE 'TENS' UNIT

Chronic pain is one of the most difficult 'conditions' to treat. Family doctors may find it frustrating as they exhaust their armoury of medication without making any significant progress on alleviating their patients' pain. The patient too becomes frustrated and, if the pain is persistent, they can begin to develop signs of anxiety and stress.

Long-term pain sufferers often turn to complementary therapies and non-prescription remedies in their search for a solution to the misery of prolonged pain. You may have seen the many newspaper and magazine advertisements which offer 'pain relief without drugs'. This may be achieved through using Transcutaneous Electrical Nerve Stimulation, ('TENS').

IMPROVING INFORMATION

TENS can be very effective in treating both chronic and acute pain. However, it is not a case of simply applying electrodes and switching on the machine. Many people who have tried TENS unsuccessfully needed only a few simple instructions on how to use the device properly in order to achieve the results they were looking for. Unfortunately, there are very few instruction books supplied with TENS units which cover the subject adequately. In addition, some clinicians are poorly informed about how to get the most from TENS units and consequently inaccurate information may be passed to patients.

This booklet addresses the problem of insufficient or inaccurate information. Designed to be easily understood without prior medical knowledge, it explains what pain is and how TENS can help, offers guidance on the positioning for the electrodes, suggests how to select the most suitable machine and includes advice on operating and adjusting the unit to maximise its effectiveness.

ABOUT THIS BOOK

Take some time to read through all of this book carefully and follow the steps given as a plan of action. You will find that TENS will not cure your pain, but it should make life tolerable again. The clinic where I practiced has carried out many studies in the effectiveness of TENS and 80% of users report significant benefit from using it. All of these people received regular instruction on how to position the electrodes and adjust their machine correctly. To achieve the same results, you should follow the instructions in this manual accurately.

I have attempted to keep the text concise in order to encourage you to read and reread the contents. If the subject was simple, this book wouldn't be necessary but be patient - remember that the best person to treat your pain with TENS is YOU! Don't be tempted to skip parts of the book; you will only obtain the best performance from your machine if you understand fully how TENS interacts with the nervous system and pain.

MEASURING PAIN

Measuring pain is an essential part of managing it. Pre-treatment levels are required to assess the most effective method of treatment so before you move on to the next page, you should use the following guide to gauge your level of pain and write down your pain score.

Imagine that a score of '0' represents no pain at all and a score of '10' is the worst pain imaginable. Write down the number from 1 to 10 that best describes your pain (a) at its MOST in a single week, and (b) at its LEAST in a single week.

If you find it difficult to imagine your pain in these terms, try drawing a straight line of 10 cm. Write 'least pain' at one end and 'worst pain' at the other and mark the line at the point you consider reflects the strength of your pain at its most in a week and its least in a week. You can now take a ruler and measure the distance from the point marked 'least pain' to the mark which represents your pain level and note down the number in centimetres.

You can also make a note of how far and for how long you can comfortably walk or perform some other form of activity which is affected by your pain, eg. vacuuming, driving, ironing etc.

Put these scores on one side for the moment. We'll return to them once we've used the TENS machine.

What is pain?
and how can TENS affect it?

TYPES OF PAIN

Pain is usually a warning that something is wrong with our body - it's an urgent message to prevent us from damaging our tissue further. We often respond to new or **acute pain** by withdrawing our hand or foot from the danger in order to limit the damage it will cause. If, for example, we were to twist an ankle, the pain would prevent us from running and if the ankle were to be badly sprained, even walking would be inhibited. This acute pain limits use of the damaged ankle until the injury has had time to heal sufficiently and so acute pain as a symptom of injury is actually beneficial.

Under normal circumstances, as the damaged tissue repairs itself, the pain gradually lessens until we are no longer aware of it and can continue walking, running etc. quite normally. However, there are occasions when pain continues beyond the time taken for tissue to heal. When this occurs, the pain is no longer a symptom but a problem in its own right. This type of pain is referred to as **chronic pain**. It is not necessary to have suffered an injury to experience chronic pain - it may even arise following 'successful' surgery. This 'untreatable' pain is sometimes associated with diseases such as arthritis or simple wear and tear of the body.

From a medical point of view, pain doesn't show up on x-rays, ultrasound scans or even Magnetic Resonance Imaging (MRI). Without any physical evidence, both patient and doctor can suspect that the pain is actually imagined.

HOW DO WE FEEL PAIN?

The pain message is transmitted from the injured area via some of the smallest of the body's nerve fibres to the spinal cord and then on to the brain which translates the messages and makes us 'feel' the pain. The painful sensations are 'remoted' to the injured area so that if we burn our hand, we quickly withdraw the hand rather than pulling back our head.

There are millions upon millions of small nerve fibres throughout the body and it only requires five impulses a second in five nerve cells to produce chronic pain. Imagine then how difficult it can be to trace the source of a patient's chronic pain - it makes the search for the Holy Grail look a soft option in comparison!

LARGE DIAMETER NERVE FIBRES

In addition to the small nerve fibres which allow the sensation of pain to be felt, the human body is also equipped with thicker nerve fibres. These carry less unpleasant sensations such as warmth, touch and the position of our joints, helping us to form an impression of our environment. The sensation of touch is particularly relevant when considering pain, since as we know, anywhere in the world, if someone accidentally knocks their elbow, they instinctively rub it. This rubbing action excites the larger nerve fibres which, in turn, have an effect on the transmission of signals from the smaller 'pain-carrying' nerves. It seems the benefit of stimulating greater activity in the larger nerve fibres may be threefold:

1. The speed of small nerve cell transmission is reduced
2. The amount of information transmitted from the small nerves to the spinal cord is reduced (known as the 'Pain-gate')
3. Under certain circumstances, the brain will produce its own pain-killing substance (known as endorphins or endogenous opioids)

The ancient Egyptians explored this phenomenon without understanding what was happening in the nerves. Hieroglyphics discovered, illustrate a practice of standing sufferers of painful gout on electric eels. We may be better athletes today, but performing a balancing act on a slippery eel would still be beyond most of us!

In 1969, the scientists Melzack and Wall described something called the 'Pain-gate' (see point 2 above). The theory of the pain gate lead to the development of TENS units designed specifically to stimulate the large diameter nerve fibres.

Don't rush off and buy or try your TENS machine yet. The next section in the book explains how to select a suitable machine, how to set and operate it and where to place the electrodes. This is all essential information that you should know before proceeding to use the equipment.

The TENS Machine

IMPORTANT NOTES

YOU SHOULD NOT USE A TENS MACHINE:

- If you have a pacemaker fitted
- If you are in the first three months of pregnancy do not place electrodes on the trunk or pelvis
- If your skin is broken or fragile where the electrodes are to be placed
- Whilst driving or operating machinery
- Over insensitive skin
- If the wearer suffers from epilepsy they should not be alone when using TENS. If they suffer a seizure, the intensity may be accidentally increased thus causing skin damage

SELECTING A TENS MACHINE

There are many different types of TENS unit on the market and various sources for acquiring them. They can be purchased by mail order, via specialists shops and chemists, or directly from the manufacturer or importer of the unit.

You should be aware that some units are restricted in their scope of output combinations and consequently may limit the potential for trying various options. This can be a crucial factor in finding the best output required to control your particular pain. Be wary of fantastic claims and exaggerated lists of what the supplier says the TENS can treat.

The following guide provides a profile of the optimum TENS machine. You may not require any more from your unit, but you must not accept anything less.

1. The unit should be small enough to wear comfortably on the belt whilst on the move
2. There should be two outlets, each accepting one pair of wires. Each outlet should in turn have its own control knob to enable independent adjustment of the current. The machine should therefore drive four electrodes.
3. The unit should include features enabling you to:
   - adjust pulse width - most units will have at least 80 to 220 micro seconds variability
   - adjust pulse rate or frequency - 2 to 150 hertz allowing a gradual increase between these outputs
   - switch between 'constant' and 'burst'
   - have two separate, easily accessible intensity controls giving between 0 and 80 mA into a 500 Ohm load

Don't worry if you don't understand the above - all will become clear as you read on. For the moment, all you need to do is continue reading and then refer to the features above when you are ready to buy a machine.

ELECTRODES

The electrodes are the flexible pads which are placed against the skin and connected to the TENS machine by thin wires which carry the current from the unit to the pads. The current then excites the underlying nerves.

There are basically two types of electrode:

- a rubber electrode which is smeared with conductive gel and held in the appropriate place with sticky tape, eg. Micropore
- self-adhesive electrodes which are pre-coated with a sticky gel which conducts electricity

Of the two types, the self-adhesive type is much easier to use, though they may be slightly more expensive. Your supplier should be able to offer you spares for both wires and electrodes as they both wear out in time.

In this manual, I will refer to 'black' and 'red' electrodes. A black electrode is known as the 'distal' electrode and is connected via the black wire to the TENS unit. The red electrode is called the 'proximal' electrode and is connected to the unit by a red wire.

You must NOT place electrodes over the front of the neck -
this can cause problems with blood pressure!

NERVES

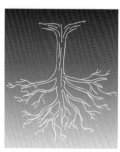

Figure 1.

If you imagine a tree without its leaves and positioned upside down, this resembles the body's nervous system, (see *Figures. 1 and 2*) The roots (now at the top) represent the brain; the trunk represents the spinal cord and the branches and twigs of the tree are like the peripheral nerves which gradually become thinner as they reach the furthest points of your limbs. The nerves are more symmetrical than the

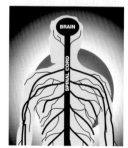

Figure 2.

random order of branches in a tree but this illustration gives you some idea of how the nervous system is structured.

Specific parts of the body are served not only by specific nerves, but each nerve has its own 'entrance' into the spinal column and then into the spinal cord. Earlier, I referred to the importance of stimulating the larger nerves in order to 'block' the painful impulses in the smaller nerves. The fact that the two belong to the same group is critical. If your pain is deduced as being carried along the sciatic nerve for example, then this is the nerve which should be stimulated with the TENS unit and hence one of the black electrodes should be placed at some point along the length of this nerve.

NERVE ROOTS

Before explaining where to place the second electrode, I should describe what a nerve root is. *Figure 3* shows part of the spinal cord viewed from behind. If you feel one of the bony vertebra that lay under the skin running down the centre of your neck or back and then move your finger a couple of centimetres to the left or right, your finger will now be over the nerve root for that level of your spine. The nerve root is the first part of the nerve just outside the spinal cord. There are eight pairs of nerve roots

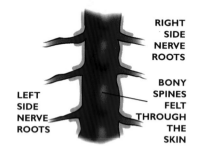

Figure 3. *Spinal Cord from behind*

in the neck (or cervical region), twelve pairs in the upper back (or thoracic region), five pairs in the lower back (or lumbar region), and five pairs in the pelvic (or sacral) area.

Returning to the example of the sciatic nerve, a suitable place for the red electrode may be over one of the nerve roots which serves this particular nerve. Note that there are two nerve roots at each level of the spine, one entering from the left and the other from the right. If you had placed the first electrode on your left leg, then the second electrode must be placed over the nerve root on the same side. This will all become clearer as you read on.

DERMATOMES

A dermatome describes an area of the skin which is served by a single nerve root. As most of us are constructed in more or less the same way, anatomists have mapped out a body diagram of where the dermatomes are positioned across the body. The illustrations on page 13-15 show the location of the dermatomes. These maps will assist us later when deciding where to place the electrodes to treat your pain.

UNDERSTANDING DERMATOMES

Each nerve root serves a known area of the skin. This area is not exclusive - there is no fine line separating the borders between dermatomes but rather, each area contains a certain amount of overlap across adjacent areas. The dermatomes are named after the nerve root which serves it and the following table describes how the dermatomes are designated.

C1 to C8	Neck or cervical spine
T1 to T12	Chest or thorax
L1 to L5	Lower back or lumbar spine
S1 to S5	Pelvis or sacrum

If your pain does not radiate into one of the limbs and is confined to the spine, you may not need to know the dermatomes. For information on where to place the electrodes for spine pain, see page 17.

If a major part of your pain is located away from the spine, for example, down the back of your leg, you must be able to identify and find the nerve root that serves this area so that you can place the red electrode in the correct position. The black electrode, as you will remember, is placed at a point along the length of the nerve between the spine and the pain, usually just on the spinal side of the pain and sometimes directly over it.

Placing the black (distal) electrode is relatively easy - you are guided by your pain. To place the red (proximal) electrode, you must first identify the dermatome associated with your pain. Use the illustrations on pages 13-15 to locate the area in which the pain is felt and write down the letter and number corresponding to the dermatome identified for this area. We now need to find the appropriate vertebra alongside which you will place the red electrode. Thankfully, rather like the pubs that people use to describe a route when giving directions, there are a few landmarks to guide us.

LOCATING THE VERTEBRAE

The Neck
If you drop your chin towards your chest, a lump will rise in the middle of the back of your neck, almost level with your shoulders. This is C7. Count the vertebrae up from this to find the one you need and you will locate the desired nerve root.

The Chest
T1 is the next vertebra below C7. If you place your arms by your sides and ask someone to find the vertebra which lies midway between the lowest points of your shoulder blades, this vertebra is T7. Again, you can count up from T7 or down from T1 to locate the desired vertebra and nerve root. In practice, if your pain is on the front or side of your chest, place the black electrode over the pain, or at the spinal side of the pain. Then follow the rib line to the spine and place the red electrode alongside the spine.

The Lower Back
Place your hands on your hips and feel firmly up and down until you locate the upper-most brim of the pelvis. The vertebra in the middle of the back between these two points is L4. Count upwards to find vertebrae L3 to L1 or down one vertebra to locate L5.

Don't be too concerned if you have difficulty finding the vertebrae - it soon becomes second nature. With practice, you will be able to place your electrodes with skill and sound reason. It is important to remember that this is YOUR PAIN and that it's in YOUR INTEREST to get it right. If the electrodes are placed incorrectly, the wrong nerves will be treated and the maximum possible benefit may not be achieved.

At the back of the book, (pages 24 - 33) there are a number of 'body charts' showing examples for the most common problems of pain with some suggested electrode positions.

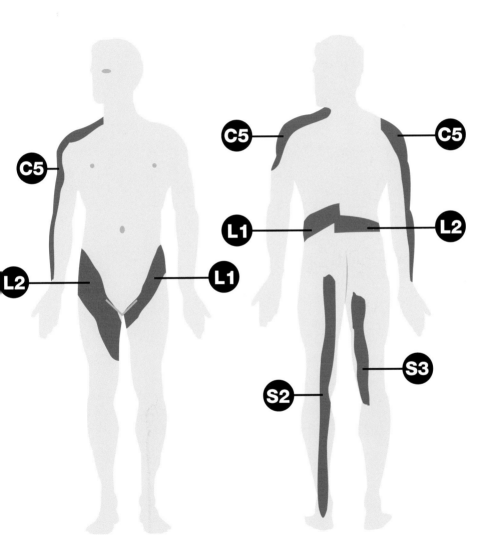

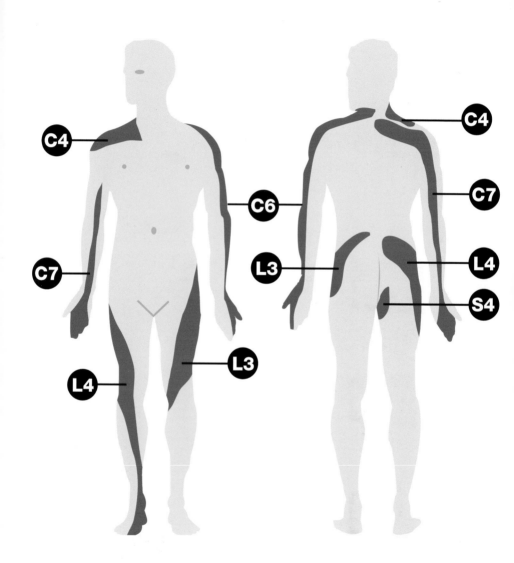

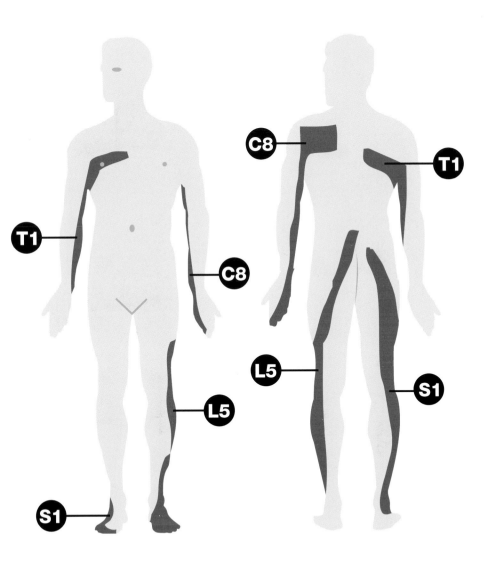

Using the TENS Machine

We now need a plan to follow - a logical progression in setting and then adjusting the TENS machine. Don't forget that we are not looking for a miracle cure, but a significant reduction in pain. Temporary analgesia is probably the best way to describe a good result.

The first part of this book described how stimulating the large nerves affected the transmission of the small, pain-carrying nerves. How you set the machine will determine whether pain is managed by 'pain-gating' (reducing the amount of painful impulses transmitted by the spinal cord to the brain) or by encouraging the brain to produce the natural painkillers - endorphins.

Figure 4..shows a typical unit and the available adjustment options. If your machine is different to the example shown, examine the instructions that accompanied the machine that you are using in order to identify the position of each switch.

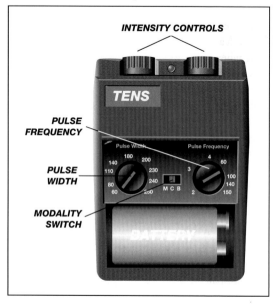

Figure 4. A typical TENS unit

The first, and usually the most successful method of pain control is that which stimulates pain-gating. It requires the following setting on your TENS unit:

> **1.** Set the Pulse Width to 200 microseconds
> **2.** Set the Modality switch to 'C' or CONSTANT or if your machine is marked 'N' for NORMAL, use this setting. (There will usually be Burst and Modulated options too)
> **3.** Set the Frequency (or Pulse Rate) to 80 Hz

Set your machine as described above. The next stage is to decide where to place the electrodes.

POSITIONING THE ELECTRODES

Refer back to the illustrations of dermatomes on pages 13-15. Remember that these are the areas of the skin which are supplied by certain nerve roots. Locate the correct dermatome by marking the picture carefully at the point where your main pain is felt. This will help to guide you when positioning the electrodes.

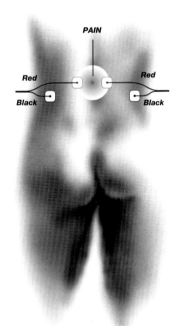

As a general guide, the electrode connected to the red lead should be placed alongside the spine where the dermatome (on which your pain lies) enters/exits the spine. (see *Figure 2*). The electrode connected to the black lead should be placed either directly over your pain or closer to the spine within the dermatome where the pain is felt. Make sure that both electrodes are placed on the same side of your body and that the electrodes are not connected to the machine at this stage.

If your pain is felt on both sides of the body, you will need to use both sets of leads and four electrodes - one pair on the left and the

Figure 5. Electrode Positions for Controlling Lower Back Pain

other pair on the right. If your pain is in the middle of your back, you will also need to use both pairs of electrodes in the position shown in *Figure 5*.

SWITCHING ON

Once the electrodes are correctly positioned with the lead connected to each one, you are then ready to connect them to the unit. Make sure that the unit is switched off before doing this.

After checking that the unit settings are as described on page 16, you can switch the unit on. Increase the intensity control until you can feel a strong but comfortable tingling sensation under at least one of each pair of electrodes. If you can feel a tingle under both electrodes of the pair or pairs being used, this is acceptable but not necessary for pain control.

Congratulations! You have now taken the first step in taking charge of your pain.

A DAILY ROUTINE

Continue to take all of your medication for the moment. If you have good results using the TENS machine, you may be able to reduce your medication in the future. You should discuss this with your doctor after about one month of using TENS.

Whilst using TENS, your day should follow the routine described below:

* Before positioning the electrodes in the morning, you must wash and dry your skin. If you shower or bathe in the mornings, there is no need for further skin cleaning. This practice ensures a good electrical contact, extends the life of the electrodes and reduces the risk of skin irritation.

* Place the electrodes in the correct positions.

* Switch your machine on and adjust the intensity control until you feel a comfortable tingle. DON'T be tempted to turn the intensity up too high, as this may stimulate the small nerves and make your pain worse!

* After 20 minutes or so, you may find that the tingling sensation has gone. If this is the case, gradually increase the intensity until you can feel a comfortable tingle again.

* Continue with your machine switched on for a total of 1-1^1/$_2$ hours. Each 1-1^1/$_2$ hour session constitutes a treatment. You may consider leaving the electrodes in place between treatments. Many people can tolerate this. However, if you experience skin irritation, remove the electrodes after each treatment.

* Repeat the 1-1^1/$_2$ hour treatments four times each day. This will administer a total maximum daily treatment of six hours. Choose the times to coincide with your periods of activity or 'worst pain'. If you have a problem sleeping due to your pain, try to save one of your treatments for the hour and a half before you go to bed.

* Before going to bed, remove the electrodes and place them back onto the plastic or paper backing that they were supplied with. Read the instructions that accompanied the TENS electrodes, as some manufacturers recommend storing the electrodes in a refrigerator overnight.

* Continue with the above routine for at least one week unless you experience any problems during treatment. After one week, re-score your pain to assess how effective the TENS is managing it.

WHAT TO EXPECT

After using your machine for about 20 minutes, your pain should gradually lessen. Don't expect it to disappear completely or you may be disappointed. Of the 450 people seen each year in the clinic where I worked, only 3 or 4 experienced complete resolution of their pain whereas 80% experienced a significant reduction in their pain. This allows them to live a much fuller life as a result.

After switching off the TENS, your pain will steadily return over a variable period of time - this is known as 'carry-over'. Depending on the individual, the carry-over period may last for anything from minutes to days. You may feel that the pain is not as severe when it begins to return but unless you continue to apply regular stimulation with your TENS, it may eventually return to its former glory. If the carry-over period is significantly long, then TENS treatments may be reduced to every other day.

Don't forget to return to the pain scoring technique described on page 5 in order to assess the effectiveness of the treatment. Do this before looking at the score you gave a week ago, then compare the two scores. Is it better, worse or still the same? If the pain score is halved during the use of TENS, this is considered a good result.

INCREASING ACTIVITY

Effective TENS treatments will provide you with a 'window' in which your pain is more tolerable. Don't be afraid to **slowly** increase your activity during these periods. Remember the difference between acute and chronic pain - acute pain is designed to prevent movement during healing whereas in chronic pain syndromes, all healing has taken place. It is natural to be cautious of becoming more active, but fear of movement will cause you more problems than movement itself.

THE ENDORPHIN ALTERNATIVE

If, after a week of using the TENS regularly, where you have faithfully followed the instructions on the preceding pages, you do not experience good pain management, it may be necessary to try managing the pain using endorphin production, (see point 3 of the table on page 7). This will require adjustment of your TENS unit as follows: (Remember to disconnect the unit from the electrode wires before adjusting the settings)

> **1.** Leave the Pulse Width setting at 200 microseconds
> **2.** Set the Modality switch to 'B' or BURST
> **3.** Increase the Frequency (or Pulse Rate) to 100 Hz

At the above settings, you will find the sensation 'pulsing' rather than the 'tingling' that you have experienced so far. On some machines, the lights may also pulsate.

Using the machine on its new settings, you should follow the same course as previously described, ie. 4 times a day for 1-1¹/₂ hours each time. Again, continue treatments for a week before you make further adjustments, unless problems arise.

After one week, re-score your pain again and compare the score with that taken before TENS treatments began and with that taken after using TENS on the 'constant' or 'normal' setting. Don't forget that even with TENS, you will still experience good and bad days - be sure to record the **average** score.

There is an exception to using only low intensities of stimulation. If you have not achieved pain management on the 'Burst' setting so far, leave your machine on the Burst setting but increase the intensity until you can see a muscle twitch under the black (distal) electrode. Continue with this level of stimulation for **TWENTY TO THIRTY MINUTES**. Repeat this treatment three times per day, giving a total treatment time of between one hour and one hour and a half per day.
This is not the most comfortable treatments but it can sometimes prove very effective.

Is your TENS more effective with the new settings? If the answer is 'yes', continue with the plan using the new settings. If the answer is 'no', return to the constant modality setting that you started with and explore low and high frequencies using the instructions on the following page.

EXPLORING LOW and HIGH FREQUENCIES

1. Leave the Pulse Width setting at 200 microseconds
2. Set the Modality switch to 'C' or CONSTANT or if your machine is marked 'N' for NORMAL, use this setting
3. Set the Frequency (or Pulse Rate) to 50 Hz for 4 days. If a good result is achieved, continue to use the machine at this setting. If not, try resetting the frequency to between 4-30Hz for the next three days.

Try using your TENS on the above settings for a week and then reassess the pain score again. If you are still not achieving reasonable pain management:
Change the Frequency (or Pulse Rate) to 120 or 150 Hz for 1 week and then reassess.

COMMON FACTORS
WHICH AFFECT GOOD PAIN MANAGEMENT

• Incorrect positioning of electrodes. Even if you start with them in the right place, you must replace them **accurately** each time that you use them.

• Not using the TENS for the correct periods. Remember that treatments should last for 1-1¹/₂ hours and be carried out 4 times each day.

• Turning up the machine's intensity too high.

• Returning to activity too quickly. Good pain management depends on you returning to activity **slowly**.

• Caffine: Research has indicated that the amount of caffine found in 2-3 cups of coffee may be sufficient to block the pain relieving effects of TENS. This may not apply to decaffinated tea and coffee.

Some Common Problems

SKIN REACTION UNDER THE ELECTRODES

- Leaving your TENS on for too long can result in over-stimulation. Allow the skin to heal and use TENS only for the periods described.

- Turning your TENS too high can cause skin problems. Allow the skin to heal and use TENS at a lower intensity.

- Some people experience an allergic reaction to the adhesive coating on the surface of the electrodes. Try using a different make of electrode if you suspect that this is the cause of the problem.

- If you continue to experience skin problems, you may try reducing the Pulse Width setting to 150 microseconds or even 100 microseconds if problems persist.
  This option is only effective if your pain is also reduced at the new lower setting.

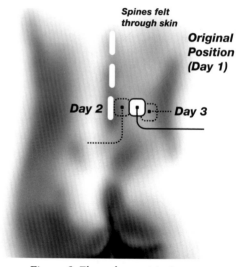

- Alternatively, move the electrode position each day by just the width of the electrode. You must ensure that the electrode is still positioned over the appropriate dermatome. (see *Figure 6*)

Figure 6. Electrode repositioning

- You may find it necessary to remove the electrodes after each treatment to allow the skin to recover.

ELECTRODES WON'T STICK

- **Oily skin.** Try thoroughly cleansing the skin with soap and water then rinse and dry the area well around the electrode sites. If this doesn't help, try cleansing the skin with a swab impregnated with alcohol. As a last resort, hold the electrode in place using a sticky tape such as Mircopore.

- **Hairy skin.** Clip away the hairs around the location of the electrode with scissors. Don't shave the area!

- **Perspiration.** The adhesive used on electrodes is water-based. If it becomes saturated, it will lose its adhesive qualities. Instead of placing the electrodes on the plastic film before going to bed, try leaving them face up overnight to allow them to dry out. Alternatively, equip yourself with two sets of electrodes and use one set for one day and the other the next.

- **Electrodes too dry.** As the electrode's adhesive is water-based, if they become too dry they can lose their adhesiveness. Before you go to bed, moisten the adhesive surface with just a few drops of water and place the moistened electrodes on the plastic backing overnight.

- **Wear and tear.** Eventually, your electrodes will wear out and require replacement. You can reasonably expect them to last for 4 to 12 weeks, depending on your skin type.

HEADACHES

TENS on certain settings will stimulate the production of endorphins. Even though these molecules have a role in reducing pain, they can sometimes cause a 'hangover' headache. If this can be avoided by changing the TENS settings to one of those previously described without affecting your pain management, continue with this course of action. If you are so sensitive to TENS that you suffer headaches on each of the alternative settings, you may reduce the Pulse Width control. Try 150 microseconds and if this does not help, reduce the Pulse Width to 100 microseconds. Again, this solution is only of value if your pain remains controlled on the new setting.

Central Neck Pain
Without Pain Radiating to the Arm

In each of the following ten examples, the radiated pain has been illustrated on the left side of the body, simply for the sake of clarity. If your radiated pain is on the right side of your body, the electrodes should be placed in a 'mirror image' of those shown here. Hold the picture up to a mirror and you will see clearly where to position your electrodes.

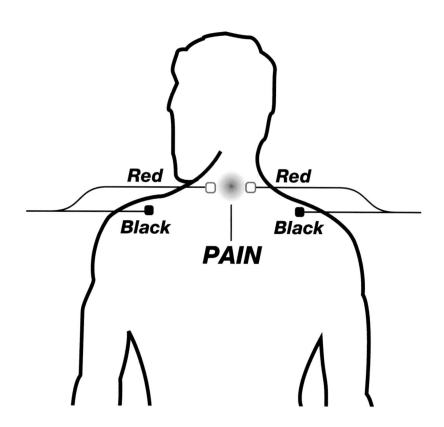

Central Neck Pain
With Pain Radiating to the Shoulder (*left shown*)

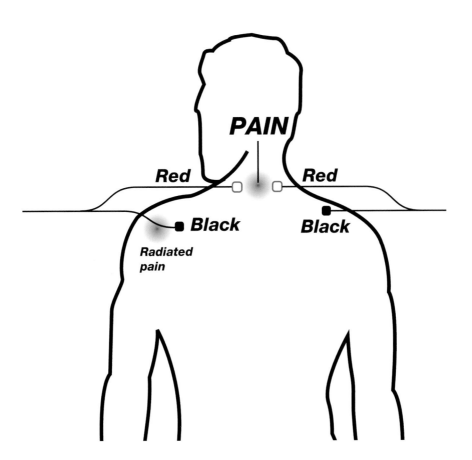

PAIN

Red

Red

Black

Black

Radiated
pain

Central Neck Pain
With Pain Radiating to the Back of the Arm (*left shown*)

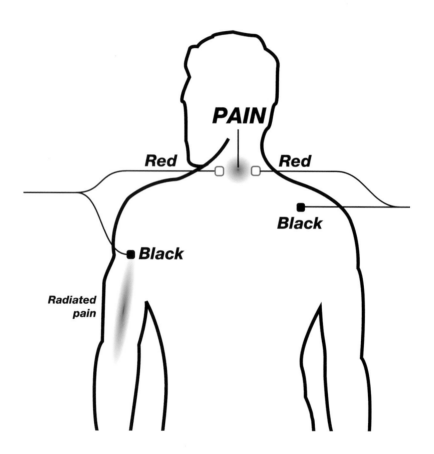

Central Neck Pain
With Pain Radiating to the Front of the Arm

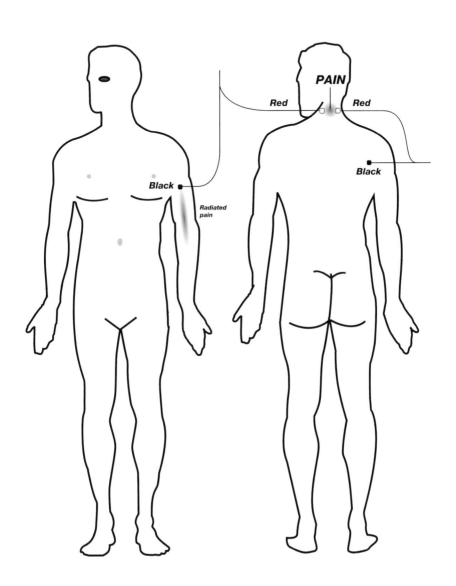

Shoulder Pain
Without Central Neck Pain

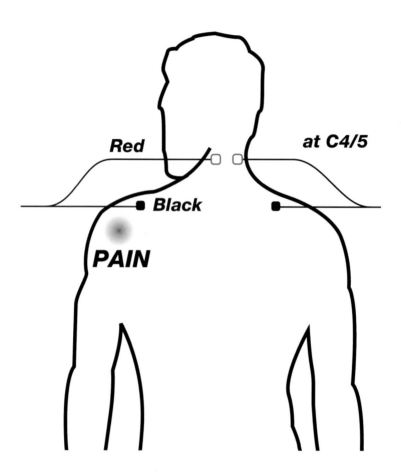

Red

at C4/5

Black

PAIN

Remember that TENS works by affecting the nerves and spinal cord. The red electrode is still placed alongside the spine.

Chest Wall Pain

due to i) injury, ii) post surgery, iii) post herpatic neuralgia (shingles)

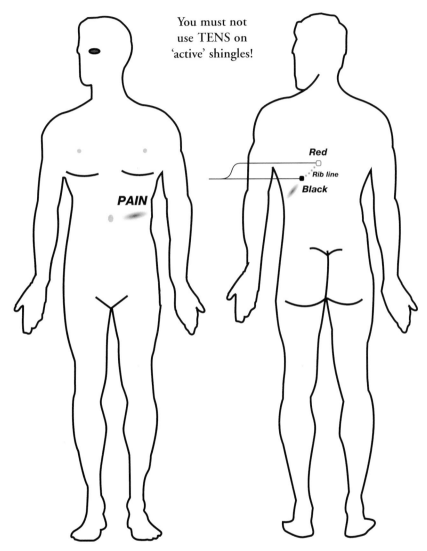

You must not use TENS on 'active' shingles!

PAIN

Red

Rib line

Black

Try first placing the black electrode close to the pain at the spine side, or if necessary, place it directly over the pain. Then follow the space between the ribs to the spine. Place the red electrode alongside the spine at that level.

Low Back Pain
Without Pain Radiating to other areas

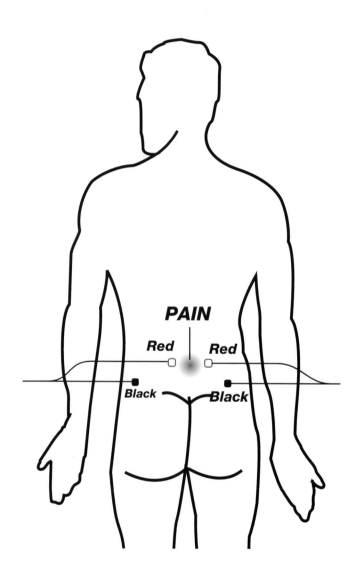

Low Back Pain
With Pain Radiating to the Buttock

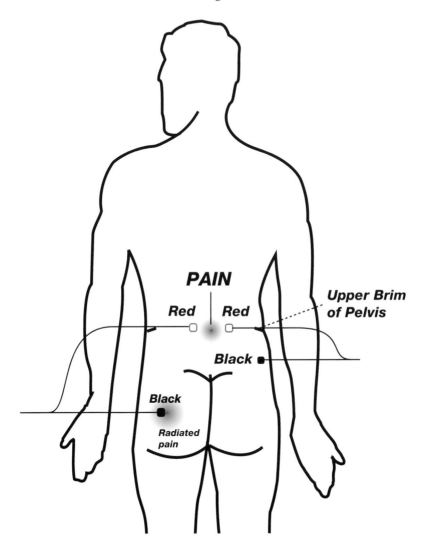

You may need to move the red electrode up or down a couple of vertebrae until you achieve good pain management.

Central Back Pain
With Pain Radiating to the Leg

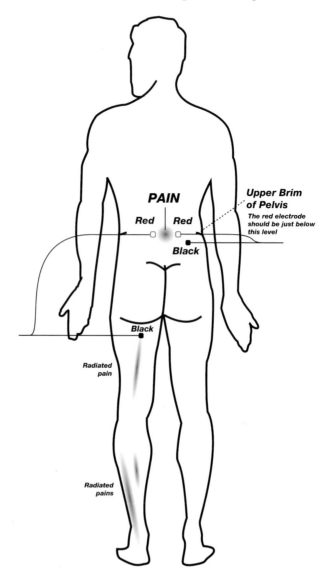

These electrode positions will also serve where pain is radiated to the back or side of the calf.

Low Back Pain
With Pain Radiating to the Front of the Leg

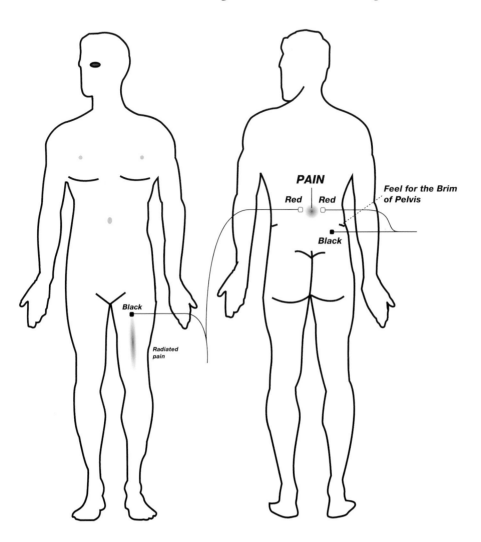

When pain is radiated to the front of the leg, L1, L2 or L3 may be the responsible level. You may find it necessary to move the red electrode up or down a vertebra to achieve good pain management.

Nausea

The causes of nausea can be varied and may be the result of an anaesthetic, certain medications or that seen in the early stages of pregnancy.

TENS can be used to treat nausea by placing the black electrodes over a very easily found acupuncture point. This point is called Circulation 6 and is described below.

If you turn your hand palm up you will notice that there are two or three skin creases where the wrist bends. Place the black electrode so that its centre is approximately two inches above the middle of the crease which is closest to the hand (see below).

The Red electrode may be placed over the same surface of the forearm - six inches higher or over the fleshy part of the hand just below the thumb.

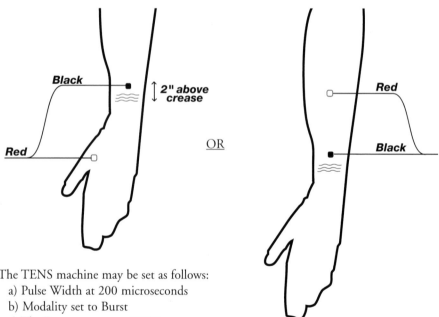

The TENS machine may be set as follows:
  a) Pulse Width at 200 microseconds
  b) Modality set to Burst
  c) The Frequency set to 100Hz

Stimulate for between five minutes and one hour. Repeat as often as necessary to control the nausea. Try to leave at least one hour between treatments.

If the above settings do not help, try the following:
  a) Pulse Width at 200 microseconds
  b) Modality set to Constant
  c) The Frequency set to 10-15Hz

Stimulate for five minutes every two hours.

Migraine and Headaches

There are several acupunture points that are used by clinicians to treat migraine. There is one which is easily located and often produces positive effects when stimulated with TENS. The point is called Colon 4 and is located on the hand (see below).

If you allow the thumb to lie against the hand, the soft tissue on the back of the hand between the base of the index finger and the wrist rises. The highest point of this 'mound' is Colon 4.

If you place your thumb from the other hand over this high point and then press firmly, you will find that this point is often tender to deep pressure just before, during and after headaches or migraine. This is the point over which you must place the black electrode. Place the electrodes on the side that displays the greatest degree of tenderness.

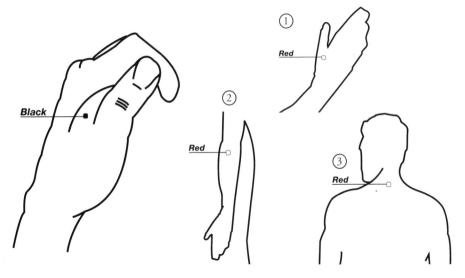

There are several sites where the red electrode may be placed.
Try each to discover which works best for you.

1) On the palm of the hand there is a fleshy pad at the base of the thumb
2) On the back of the forearm just below the elbow on the highest point of the muscle
3) Alongside the spine adjacent to the vertebra C6 on the same side as the black electrode

Set the TENS to Burst, 100Hz with a Pulse Width of 200 microseconds. Stimulate for up to one and a half hours. Repeat up to four times daily. If this is not successful, try Constant, 80-100Hz.

Stimulating one side only, often is sufficient to effect the pain. However, if a significant result is not evident, try stimulating both left and right sides.

Conclusion

Each individual may require different placements for electrodes. The positions shown in this book may provide a good starting point. There may also be an occasion when positioning the electrodes each side of a painful joint can help e.g. the front and back of a painful shoulder (see below).

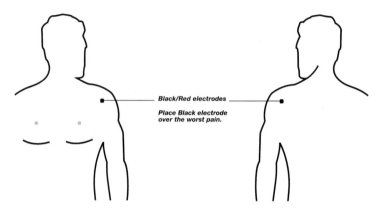

Black/Red electrodes

**Place Black electrode
over the worst pain.**

Research has shown that the direct stimulation of nerves (that have been surgically exposed) with the red lead or anode can cause blocking of the nerve impulses under the electrode. This may not be the case when surface electrodes are used. However, if you find that you are not achieving good results with the electrode positions previously described, try moving the red electrode or simply reverse the lead wires. You must remember that the black electrode is the active electrode and therefore this should lie over one of the nerve bundles serving the painful area.

Following the instructions included in this book will provide you with a good foundation for pain management with TENS. You may need to 'fine tune' the position of the electrodes as each major nerve has contributions from several nerve roots. Happily, these are grouped together so moving the red electrode up and down a vertebra will suffice. You might also consider placing electrodes over the appropriate acupuncture points if you have followed the instructions yet failed to reduce your pain.

The subject covered by this book is fascinating but if I had included everything, it would have been far too unwieldy. Do work through all the alternatives before deciding that TENS is not helping. I have seen many cases where pain management was not achieved until the last combinations were tried so persevere with your machine and stick by your routine to make the most of TENS.

Alan King